# YOUR PREGNANCY

## A SURVIVAL GUIDE

### BY MARTIN BAXENDALE

# INTRODUCTION

<u>Don't forget to whinge!</u> That is of course one of the most important things to remember about being pregnant (that, plus taking full advantage of the opportunity to constantly stuff your face with all your favourite fattening foods and blame it on the baby).

Of course you need to plan and prepare, to practice and learn stuff, share all the happy moments and support one another through the difficult bits, blah, blah, blah…..

And yes, pregnancy can be an exciting and thrilling adventure. But it can also be bloody hard work, what with morning sickness, backaches, and all that.

So let's face it, you'll never get a better excuse to have a good whinge, and the best bit is, no-one can say a word about it. And even if they do, the rules say you get to bite their heads off, and no-one can say a word about that either.

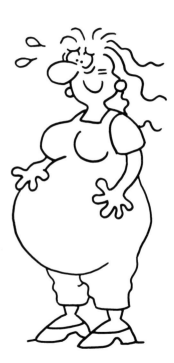

# MAIN PREGNANCY COMPLAINTS

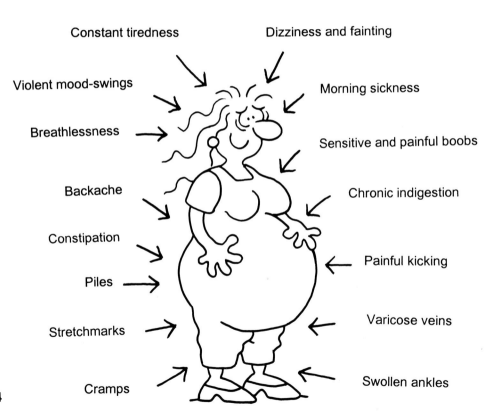

Constant tiredness

Dizziness and fainting

Violent mood-swings

Morning sickness

Breathlessness

Sensitive and painful boobs

Backache

Chronic indigestion

Constipation

Piles

Painful kicking

Stretchmarks

Varicose veins

Cramps

Swollen ankles

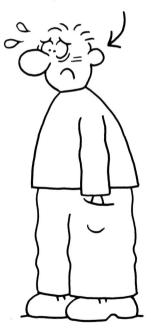

Not allowed to touch incredibly large but very sensitive and painful boobs.

# COPING DURING PREGNANCY

## MORNING SICKNESS

You may experience this in the early stages of your pregnancy. If so, try to snack through the day, eating little and often rather than large meals.

Also, avoid greasy and very strong-flavoured foods that might bring on the nausea, such as fish-and-chips, cheese-burgers, fried liver and onions, pickled herring, smoked mackerel, kippers, ripe French cheeses that smell like pongy feet...oops! Sorry! Breathe slowly and wait for it to pass. Maybe a glass of water will help.

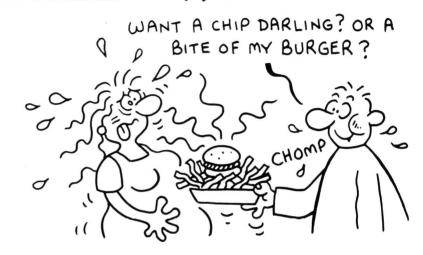

WANT A CHIP DARLING? OR A BITE OF MY BURGER?

CHOMP

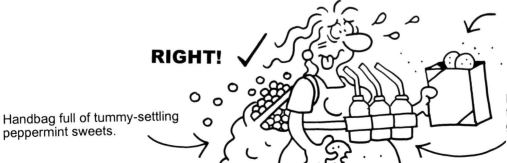

**RIGHT!** ✓

Handbag full of tummy-settling peppermint sweets.

Dry plain crackers for munching when queasy.

Drinking bottles filled with tummy-settling peppermint, ginger and camomile teas.

5

# STRETCHMARKS

Short of strapping yourself into a very tightly-laced corset for the duration of the pregnancy, to stop yourself from expanding (which we definitely would <u>not</u> recommend) there isn't much you can do except try the available anti-stretchmark creams and hope that they'll at least reduce the problem if not totally prevent it.

The important thing about creams is that you should use them <u>regularly</u> and <u>liberally</u> for maximum effect, so we would strongly recommend the following application measures:

**APPLYING ANTI-STRETCHMARK CREAMS :**

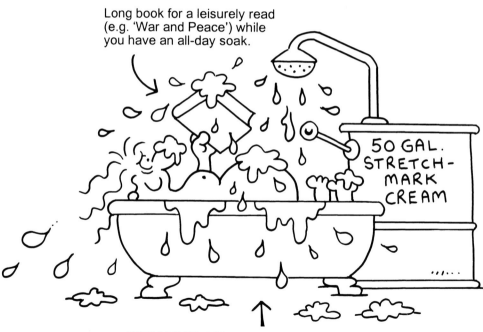

Long book for a leisurely read (e.g. 'War and Peace') while you have an all-day soak.

50 GAL. STRETCH-MARK CREAM

RECOMMENDED STANDARD APPLICATION

BEFORE GOING OUT

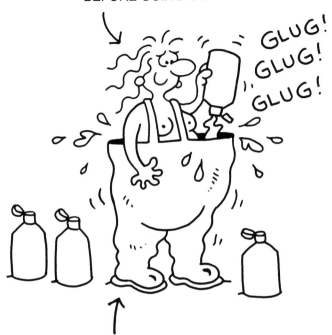

GLUG!
GLUG!
GLUG!

Full-length fisherman's rubber
waders filled with stretchmark
cream. Can be worn under baggy
dresses when out shopping etc
(though the squelching noises
as you walk may attract some
strange looks).

BEFORE GOING TO BED

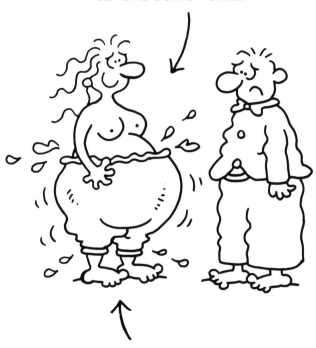

Rubber incontinence knickers
filled with stretchmark cream.

# ACHES, PAINS AND TIREDNESS

Backache, swollen ankles, breathlessness and constant tiredness are common complaints in the later stages of pregnancy, as you grow heavier and heavier.

The answer is of course to put your feet up and take things easy as much as possible. And naturally your partner will be understanding and do his utmost to give you plenty of breaks from the daily grind by doing all the shopping, cleaning, cooking etc when you need him to.

(Yeah, right! And wasn't that a flock of pigs that just flew past the window on their way south for the winter?)

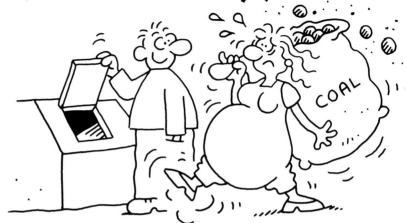

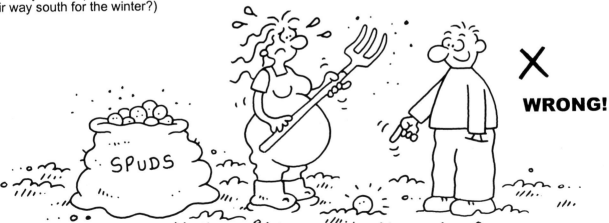

# NEEDING TO PEE ALL THE TIME

This can be a real nuisance as the baby grows larger and starts to press down on your bladder.

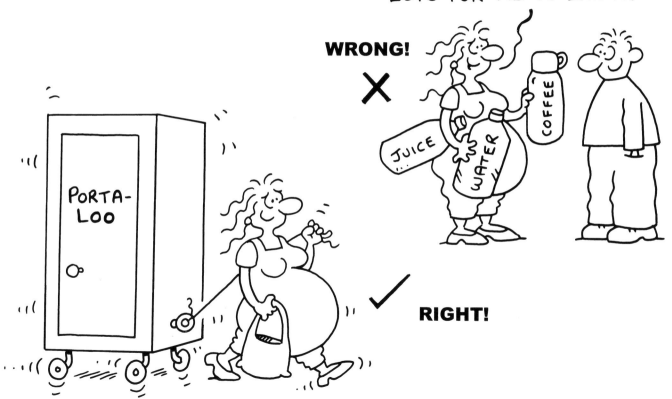

## RESTLESS NIGHTS

You may well find you have more and more restless nights as the pregnancy progresses, and especially if the baby <u>always</u> starts to kick <u>the moment you lie down</u>.

Of course some specialists claim that babies during pregnancy can't tell whether it's night or day, so they don't know they're keeping you awake. Oh yeah? Want a bet?!!

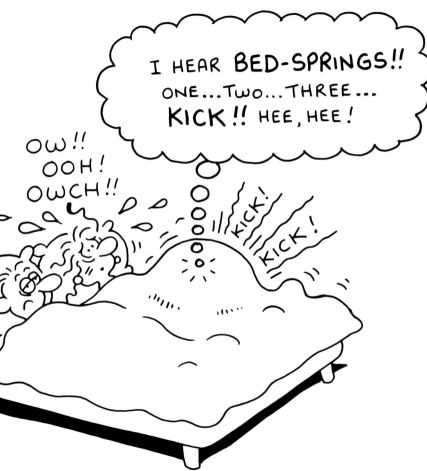

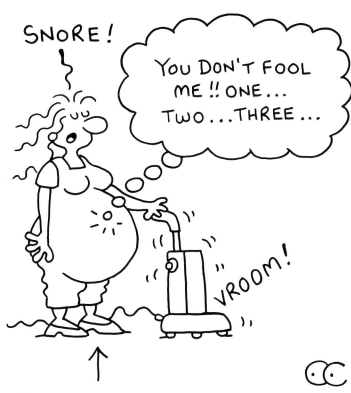

All we can suggest is that you learn to sleep <u>standing up</u>.

(The up-side to all of this is that your partner is probably just as sleepless while you're tossing and turning, most likely living in mortal fear that you'll roll over and crush him to death).

## FEELING BIG AND UNATTRACTIVE

Towards the end of the pregnancy, many women start to feel pretty much like a beached whale and may even begin to think that they're hideously huge and unattractive.

Don't call the Greenpeace help-line; just remember the following simple equation:

11

# EATING FOR TWO

Later in the pregnancy, after the morning sickness has worn off, you'll probably find you're hungry all the time.

What can we say? Enjoy! It's the best excuse you'll ever get to pig out on all your favourite fattening foods without feeling the least bit guilty.

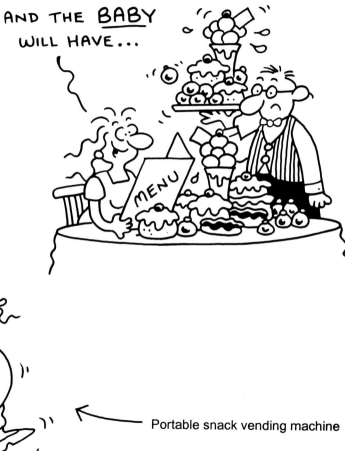

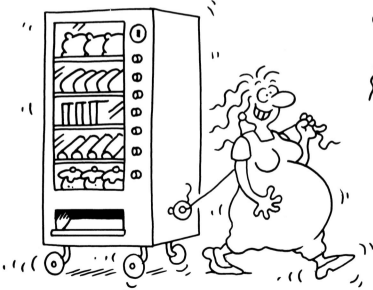

Portable snack vending machine

# SHARING THE EXPERIENCES

It's important that you share your pregnancy experiences with your partner and involve him in the whole thing as much as possible, rather than selfishly keeping it all to yourself.

Indeed, in today's caring, sharing society, your partner would probably never forgive you if you were to exclude him from any of the many amazing, wonderful and truly magical experiences of your pregnancy.

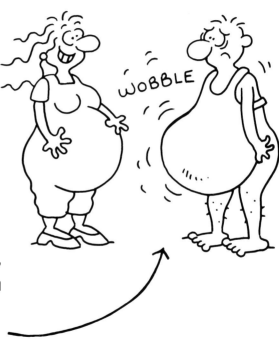

Heavy water-filled false pregnant tummy, worn under clothes for nine months to allow your partner to share the wonderful pregnancy experiences of constant backache, swollen ankles, permanent tiredness, breathlessness etc.

Add more water each month until nearly bursting, to immitate natural tummy expansion and weight increase.

Huge water-filled false pregnant boobs add still more weight and reality to your partner's exciting shared pregnancy experiences.

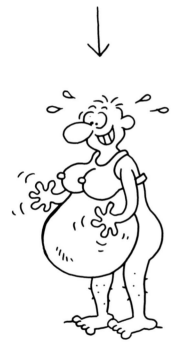

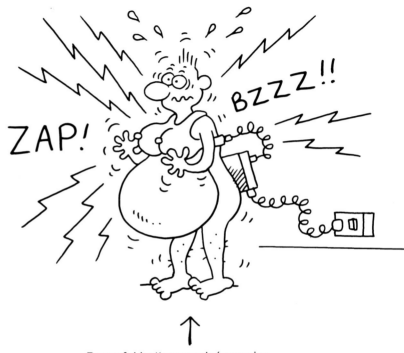

Powerful battery pack (or mains lead for indoor use) gives your partner a high-voltage shock when false boobs are squeezed, to share with your partner the incredible pregnancy experience of extremely sensitive and tender boobs.

14

To share with your partner the unique pregnancy experience of violent mood-swings throughout the day, simply mix into his favourite breakfast cereal a cocktail of as many different mind-altering drugs as you can lay your hands on.

Uppers, downers, LSD tabs, speed, etc

Cornflakes

Milk spiked with vodka

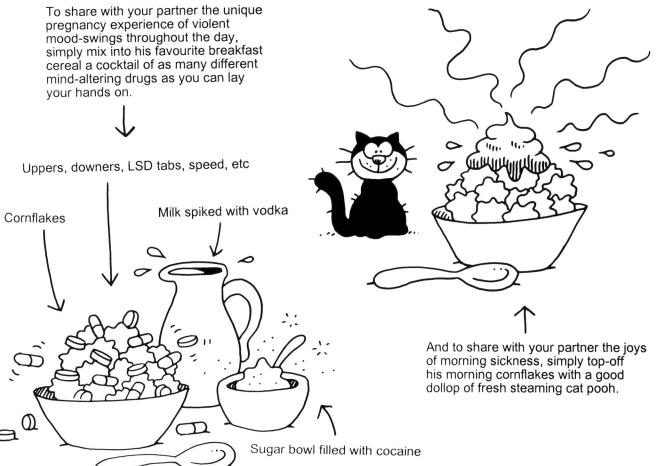

And to share with your partner the joys of morning sickness, simply top-off his morning cornflakes with a good dollop of fresh steaming cat pooh.

Sugar bowl filled with cocaine

15

Most mothers-to-be regularly talk to their babies before they're born, and playing <u>soothing music</u> for your baby during pregnancy is also highly recommended by the experts.

It's important to share this with your partner too, encouraging him to speak to the baby as well, so that baby gets used to <u>both</u> your voices, not just mummy's.

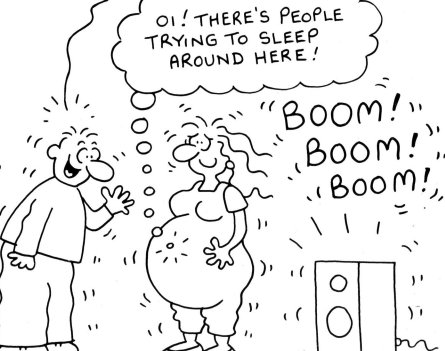

# PREPARING FOR THE BIRTH

## COMMON BIRTH PROBLEMS

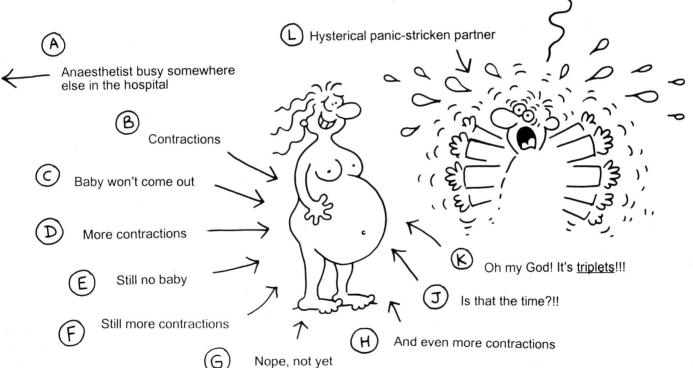

(A) Anaesthetist busy somewhere else in the hospital

(B) Contractions

(C) Baby won't come out

(D) More contractions

(E) Still no baby

(F) Still more contractions

(G) Nope, not yet

(H) And even more contractions

(J) Is that the time?!!

(K) Oh my God! It's triplets!!!

(L) Hysterical panic-stricken partner

OH MY GOD! IT WON'T COME OUT!!

## COPING WITH PANIC

No matter how much you try to prepare your partner for the birth with antenatal classes, books, videos etc, he may still panic when the time for the birth actually arrives, and especially if it goes on for more than an hour or so or becomes at all messy.

Note: try not to confuse panic over a prolonged or messy birth with your partner's normal impatience to get down the pub for a pint with the lads.

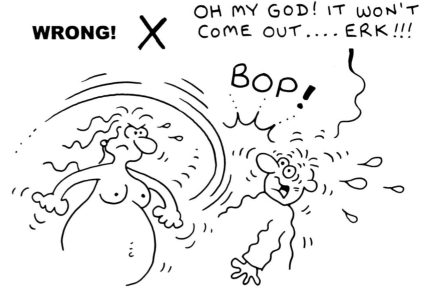

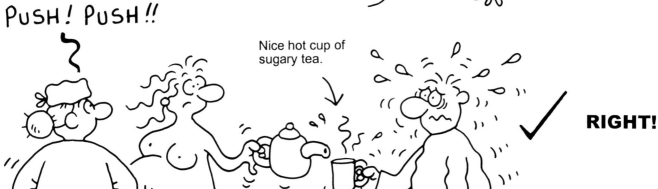

# CHOOSING THE TYPE OF BIRTH

There are various choices available when it comes to deciding exactly what type of birth you would prefer to have, including:

A) Natural birth, no drugs at all
B) Just a little gas and air
C) "Knock me out now, you bastards!"

You can also choose between a number of different birth positions, including:

A) Lying on your back
B) Kneeling on all fours or squatting
C) Floating in warm water

or, as a last resort:

D) Bouncing frantically up and down on a trampoline and screaming "Come out you little sod!!!"

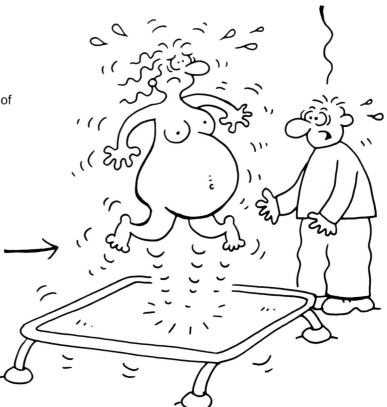

19

# PRACTISING FOR THE BIRTH

Antenatal classes, mother-and-baby books and pregnancy videos are all excellent for helping you prepare for the birth.

Yet there are one or two things they won't teach you but which are absolutely essential and should be practised regularly at home, ready for when you go into hospital:

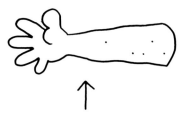

Rubber dummy hand and arm, for practising crushing your partner's fingers and gouging his arm with your fingernails while you hang frantically onto him during labour.

Repeated use in the months before the birth will build up your finger muscles for maximum finger-crushing and arm-gouging power on the day (remember also to avoid cutting your fingernails for at least a month before the birth, so they're nice and long).

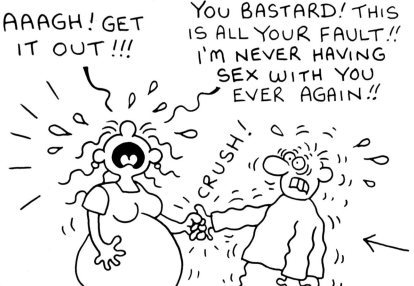

Be sure to spend plenty of time practising your birthing-room screaming, cursing and swearing as you'll naturally want to be word-perfect on the day.

# <u>REALLY</u> SHARING THE BIRTH EXPERIENCE

It's considered important these days for the father to experience the birth as well as the mother, and so fathers are generally welcomed and even expected in the birthing room.

And it's not unknown for a caring partner to have the odd mild sympathy labour pain as the mother is giving birth.

But if you <u>really</u> want your partner to share the complete joy and wonder of the birth experience with you (and why not?) then we strongly recommend the following simple procedure just before leaving for the hospital:

Ⓐ

Inflate a medium-size beach ball inside your partner's bottom.

Ⓑ  Give your partner a triple dose of a very strong laxative.

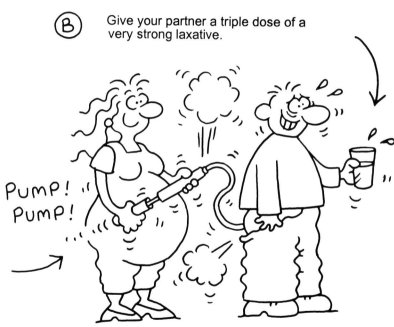

PUMP!
PUMP!

Ⓒ  Rush to hospital labour ward, having first phoned to book <u>two</u> beds.

# PREPARING FOR AFTER BABY ARRIVES

This is an essential part of your pregnancy preparations, ensuring that you have everything ready for when baby comes home, and it will inevitably take up a great deal of your time (and money) in the months leading up to the birth.

## BUYING BABY THINGS

It's important to get all the baby things that you'll need - cot, pram, nappies, feeding bottles, steriliser, clothes, dummies, etc, etc, etc - well in advance as you'll be pretty busy once baby has arrived.

For this, you will need:

A) An incredibly long bit of paper for the shopping list.
B) One self-drive articulated lorry to bring the stuff home in.
C) One fork-lift truck to unload it all.
D) A very sympathetic bank manager to provide the necessary overdraft (we recommend that you look for one with all the tell-tale signs of having a young baby of his own at home).

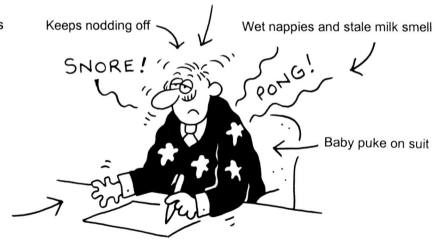

Bags under eyes from lack of sleep

Keeps nodding off

Wet nappies and stale milk smell

SNORE!

PONG!

Baby puke on suit

HOW TO RECOGNISE A SYMPATHETIC BANK MANAGER

# GETTING BABY'S ROOM READY

At first you'll probably decide to have the baby's crib or cot next to your bed, but eventually you'll want to move baby into his or her own room (unless of course you actually <u>enjoy</u> sleep deprivation).

Best to get the room ready well in advance so it'll be one less thing to worry about after baby arrives (and just in case you're not made of such strong stuff as you thought you were).

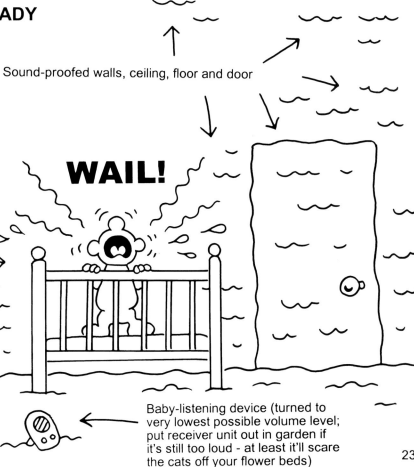

Sound-proofed walls, ceiling, floor and door

**WAIL!**

Cot

Night-light

Baby-listening device (turned to very lowest possible volume level; put receiver unit out in garden if it's still too loud - at least it'll scare the cats off your flower beds)

# PRACTISING CARING FOR BABY

You'll do plenty of this at antenatal classes, and sometimes they have lifelike new-born baby dolls for you to practise on.

However, if you want to be <u>fully</u> prepared for what it's going to be like, then we strongly recommend practising on the '<u>REALLY</u> LIFELIKE NEW-BORN BABY PRACTISE DOLL' (patent applied for).

Adjustable mouth grip for life-like breast-feeding practise: Adjusts from 'Mild pinch' through 'Vice-like clamp' to 'Oh my God! My nipple's coming off!!!'

Lifelike baby feed feature: Will automatically squirt back out at least three-quarters of every feed within a matter of seconds (special sensor will immediately recognise if you're wearing your best dress and initiate high-pressure projectile puke mode to ensure that difficult-to-clean little black number is thoroughly sprayed with milk).

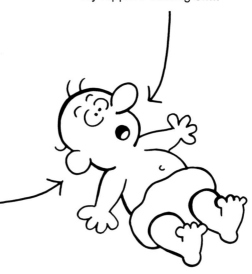

The '<u>REALLY</u> LIFELIKE NEW-BORN BABY PRACTISE DOLL' (patent applied for).

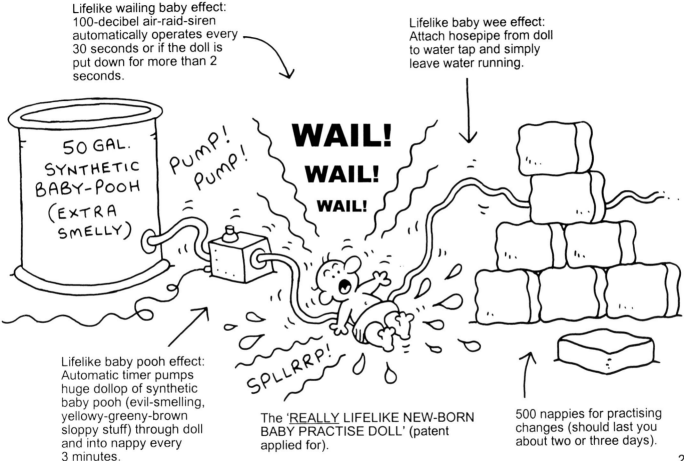

Lifelike wailing baby effect: 100-decibel air-raid-siren automatically operates every 30 seconds or if the doll is put down for more than 2 seconds.

Lifelike baby wee effect: Attach hosepipe from doll to water tap and simply leave water running.

50 GAL. SYNTHETIC BABY-POOH (EXTRA SMELLY)

PUMP! PUMP!

WAIL!
WAIL!
WAIL!

SPLLRRP!

Lifelike baby pooh effect: Automatic timer pumps huge dollop of synthetic baby pooh (evil-smelling, yellowy-greeny-brown sloppy stuff) through doll and into nappy every 3 minutes.

The 'REALLY LIFELIKE NEW-BORN BABY PRACTISE DOLL' (patent applied for).

500 nappies for practising changes (should last you about two or three days).

## PRACTISING GETTING NO SLEEP

It's best to gradually get used to sleepless nights in advance, so it doesn't come as so much of a shock to your systems when baby arrives.

Ease yourselves into it slowly, initially setting the alarm to wake you both up once or twice in the middle of the night. Then gradually increase the wake-ups until your sleep is being interrupted every hour on the hour, if not more. That should get you into the swing of it very nicely.

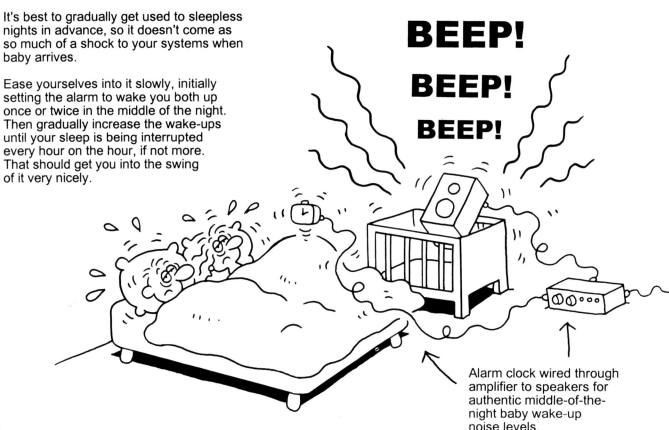

**BEEP!**

**BEEP!**

**BEEP!**

Alarm clock wired through amplifier to speakers for authentic middle-of-the-night baby wake-up noise levels.

# GETTING USED TO A SMELLY HOUSE

If you don't want to be totally overpowered by the pong after baby arrives, it's important to acclimatize yourselves gradually to the way a new baby makes the house smell.

During the pregnancy, arrange to borrow soiled nappies on a regular basis from parents in your neighbourhood who already have a new baby in the house.

Leave in a dustbin liner for a few days to mature, then scatter around your previously sweet-smelling home for that authentic "Oh my God! You've got a baby in the house!!" stench.

For fathers-to-be, this gradual acclimatization is especially important as they seem to be particularly sensitive to new baby pong, and getting daddy used to it in advance may reduce the need for him to wear breathing apparatus around the house later on.

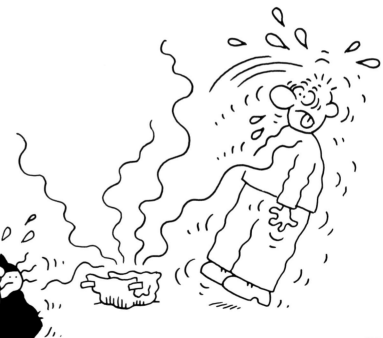

# GETTING USED TO BABY GRUNGE

Sorry, but you have to accept that everything in your previously nice clean house (furniture, carpets, curtains, walls, ceilings, pets, etc) will eventually acquire an overall grungey coating of splattered baby food, baby bogies, stale milk and baby puke.

If you're at all house-proud or the slightest bit finicky about cleanliness, we would strongly advise pre-splattering your house, so that you get acclimatized to it in advance; then hopefully at least when baby arrives you'll be so used to the mess that you won't blame it on the little darling.

If you're into home decoration and DIY, just think of it as a pre-baby home make-over. You can get some really interesting effects by sponge-stippling baby food on the walls.

Oh, and while you're pre-splattering the house with baby food etc, don't forget to do all your best clothes (especially the difficult-to-clean ones) plus the inside of the car.

Pressurized spray tank filled with sloppy baby food.

10 litre can of extra-drip satin-finish baby food.

# PRACTISING DOING EVERYTHING WITH <u>JUST ONE ARM</u>

This is an essential skill that you absolutely <u>must</u> master before baby arrives; in preparation for months and months of having to carry him or her around the house with you all the time, no matter what you're trying to do - and that includes wiping your bottom.

A bag of potatoes is about the right weight to practise with, though not as wriggly as the real thing (for that, you'd really need a small sack full of ferrets).

What's that? Can't you just <u>put the baby down</u> for a minute? Ha, ha, ha, ha, ha!! Oh, that's a good one!!! Hee, Hee, Hee!! Stop it, you're killing me!!! Get out of here!!

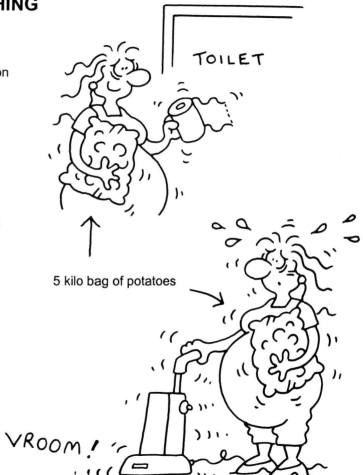

5 kilo bag of potatoes

VROOM!

29

# PRACTISING **NOT** GOING OUT

You really had better get used to this one,
and the sooner the better.

Start slowly by stopping going out with friends
to the pub, then start turning down invites to
parties, forget about the cinema and romantic
restaurant bookings, and postpone any exotic
holiday-in-the-sun plans (babies on airplanes
are a nightmare that you really don't want to
get into!)

Binned 'what's on' and restaurant guides,
cinema listings, holiday brochures, etc.

## RECOMMENDED FURTHER READING FOR NEW PARENTS:

Also from Silent But Deadly Publications, **YOUR NEW BABY - AN OWNER'S MANUAL** is an invaluable and hugely popular in-depth guide to operating, maintaining and servicing your New Baby unit, guaranteed to ensure many years of trouble-free operation.

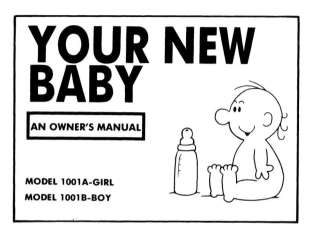

"I don't know what I would have done without your wonderful New Baby manual – I had no idea how to work my new Baby properly and thought it might be some kind of novel food-blender until I read your marvellous hand-book." (unsolicited letter from a reader, Mr. A.N. Idiot of Milton Keynes).